Not just

By the same author

Homoeopathy for the Third Age
Homoeopathy: Heart & Soul
Cure Craft

Not just a room with a Bath

*Simple and Natural Remedies for
Common Ailments that can be applied
in one's own bathroom*

DR KEITH SOUTER
DSc, MB, ChB, MRCGP, MHMA

SAFFRON WALDEN
THE C.W. DANIEL COMPANY LTD

First published in Great Britain by
The C.W. Daniel Company Limited
1 Church Path, Saffron Walden
Essex, CB10 1JP, England

Produced in association with
Book Production Consultants plc Cambridge
Typeset by Cambridge Photosetting Services
Printed and bound by St Edmundsbury Press Ltd.,
Bury St Edmunds, Suffolk

Contents

Introduction   7

SECTION ONE – THE BATH

Chapter One
The Bath in Medicine   11
Chapter Two
The Remedial Effects of Bathing   20
Chapter Three
The Bath, Shower and Basin   25
Chapter Four
Do's and Don'ts   41

SECTION TWO – THE REMEDIES

Chapter Five
Arthritis, Rheumatism & Sprains   47
Chapter Six
Skin Problems   52
Chapter Seven
Chest and Breathing Problems   57
Chapter Eight
Abdominal Problems   61
Chapter Nine
Women's Problems   67
Chapter Ten
Troublesome Infections   73
Chapter Eleven
Troubled Emotions   80

Rachel, my wife and best friend,
who makes it all worthwhile.

Introduction

There is a room in every home which is effectively a symbol of the healing Art. Unfortunately, nowadays the bathroom is merely considered a place to wash. Apart from housing the medicine cupboard it seems to have lost most of its connections with healing.

The early physicians of India, Greece and Rome all realised the healing potential of bathing. Public and private baths were considered an essential part of civilisation. Yet it was realised that it was not just the water that mattered, but the way it was used and the things which were added to it.

In the eighteenth and nineteenth centuries people flocked to the Spas of Europe to take and to bathe in the healing waters of the great centres. Naturopathic and Hydropathic hotels and clinics attracted clientele from all over the world. Then with the rapid development of orthodox Medicine in the twentieth century, hydrotherapy began to dwindle in popularity and was gradually dropped from the therapeutic armamentarium of the modern physician. Until now, that is.

Medicine goes through fashions, as does any human endeavour. In the late twentieth century as orthodoxy begins to acknowledge many of the precepts of Natural Medicine, we see that there are many ways in which the humble bath can add to improving health. Naturopathy, hydrotherapy, herbalism, aromatherapy all demonstrate the value of the bath in health care.

Arthritis and rheumatism, skin disorders, chest problems, abdominal and gynaecological conditions and various emotional troubles can all be helped by using the full potential of the bathroom. This slim volume is not meant to replace the advice of your doctor or health adviser. Its purpose is to help the individual to deal with minor health problems using very simple, natural treatments which can be applied in the comfort of one's own bathroom.

Keith Souter

SECTION ONE

THE BATH

CHAPTER ONE

The Bath in Medicine

*'The bath is useful in many diseases, in some
of them when used steadily, and in others
when not so. . . .'*

HIPPOCRATES

■ Early beginnings

Bathing is an activity which has been indulged in
by people throughout history. It has been practised for religious reasons, for pleasure and for
health purposes. People have bathed in the sea,
in rivers, lakes, springs and in an assortment of
special man-made baths.

The Bible and the Koran both contain many
references to bathing. Similarly, one of the life
goals for every Hindu is to bathe in the sacred
River Ganges. In these contexts the purpose of
bathing is very much one of purification. It is a
concept which was transformed into an ideal
when the Reverend Charles Wesley, one of the
founders of the Methodist church, preached
that 'Cleanliness is next to godliness.'

Exactly when bathing for pleasure began, no-
one knows. Yet we do have evidence that
prehistoric man constructed baths, presumably
for pleasure or health purposes. Bronze Age
tubing has been found at St Moritz in Switzer-
land at the site of natural hot springs.

One would of course expect hotter climates to
be associated with bathing for hygiene as well
as pleasure. The Minoans built great palaces
complete with rudimentary plumbed baths at
Knossos in Crete as long ago as the second
millennium BC. In addition, the homes of many

wealthy families contained personal clay bath-tubs, much like our own modern ones designed for complete immersion of the body.

This was contemporary with the early civilisations of the Indus valley, where the pre-Aryans built highly sophisticated cities at Harappa and Mohenjo-daro. These were built along a grid system, containing piped water, sewage conduits, networks of wells and both private and public baths.

The Harappa Culture, as the early Indian civilisation was known, fell to invading Aryans in about 1500BC. The synthesis of the two cultures saw the development of a new civilisation and a whole new epoch of intellectual growth. Ayurveda, the traditional system of Hindu medicine flourished, drawing upon the wisdom of the older cultures. The use of the bath was considered highly important in this new form of Medicine.

The Greeks embraced bathing as both a pleasurable and a healthy thing to do. Greek physicians extolled the virtues of different types of bath and advised upon the use of oils both in the water and for anointing before one dried off.

Hippocrates himself wrote an essay contained in his book *On Regimen in Acute Diseases*. In this he outlines both indications and contra-indications to having baths. In addition, in his famous *Aphorisms*, a series of rules and tenets of medicine, he frequently displays amazing astuteness.

For example, Aphorism V, 25:

'Swellings and pains in the joints, without ulceration, those of a gouty nature, and sprains, are generally improved by a copious affusion of cold water, which reduces the swelling, and removes the pain. . . .'

Or again, Aphorism V, 26:

'The lightest water is that which is quickly heated and quickly cooled.'

For lightest, read 'pure.' Indeed, it was not until many centuries later that it was proven that the boiling point is elevated and the freezing point drops when water contains something dissolved in it.

Greek baths were unlike the Minoan ones, however. They were designed like modern Sitz baths, whereby the bather sits rather than lies. In addition, they sometimes had facilities for water being showered down upon them from above.

In the first century BC, a Greek physician, Asclepiades of Bithynia attained great fame in Rome, where he founded the *methodical school* of medicine. He advocated using contraries (or medicines which were opposite to the illness symptoms), as well as generous diets, strenuous exercise and bathing. It is likely that this physician was largely responsible for introducing the Roman ideal of frequent baths, and indirectly responsible for the enthusiasm with which the Romans built baths near medicinal springs and wells.

As the Roman Empire spread across Europe, spas were established at Aix-le-Bains and Vichy in France (respectively called *Aquae Gratianae* and *Aquae Calidae*), and at Wiesbaden and Baden Baden in Germany (respectively *Aquae Mattiacae* and *Aurelia Aquensis*), then at Bath in England (*Aquae Sulis*).

Public baths were built in almost every Roman city and most wealthy citizens would have their own private bath. Originally Roman baths consisted of cold water baths and small pools for swimming. The Greek influence converted them to the use of hot air bathing as well, in order to open up the skin pores and induce perspiration.

It is likely that bathing was originally used to clean the skin, but the health benefits of different types of water, hot air and perspiration turned the whole activity into something both pleasurable and remedial.

The whole technological and artistic skill of the Romans was brought to bear in the construction of baths. Roman engineering invented *the hypocaust*, a system involving a suspended raised floor above heated gas chambers, which heated the room through the floor. Artists created beautiful mosaics, wall murals and filled the rooms with statuettes and fountains.

A Roman bath-house consisted of several rooms, through which the bather went in turn. The first room was called *the frigidarium*, because it was the unheated cold room where one changed. Here the bather cooled down, perhaps by having an initial cold bath or shower. After that he went to *the tepidarium*, the warm room which was the first of the rooms to receive some heat from the underfloor hypocaust. Here the bather had oils rubbed into the skin to start the process of opening the pores. After the acclimatisation had begun, he moved through to *the caldarium*, the hot room where the air was really hot and humid by virtue of a steam tank attached to the hypocaust. Indeed, so hot was this room that the floor was too hot to touch and one was obliged to wear thick wooden sandals.

In the caldarium the bather could wash his face at the central cold water *labrum*, a basin upon a pedestal, then lounge on the benches and couches and have the perspiration scraped from him with a type of smooth comb called a *strigil*. That done, he could move on to the super-hot room, *the laconicum*, before returning to the frigidarium for a further cold plunge and dry off.

■ Divinities of the bath

In most ancient cultures virtually every undertaking had a deity or divinity who would bestow his or her benevolence upon it. Very often this divinity was also associated with medicine and health.

In Ancient Egypt, Thoth the god of knowledge, writing and Medicine was considered to be the prime deity to look after the bather. After him came Bes, the Lord of Punt. He was a marriage god who looked after childbirth and the bathing of infants and women.

The Ancient Greeks invoked Hera, the wife of Zeus as a protector during bathing. Later, she was joined by Asclepius, the god of healing, and his daughter Hygeia (from whom we get the term hygiene). At the healing temples of Asclepius, bathing was considered an essential part of the treatment.

The Romans considered Minerva, the goddess of commerce, education and robust force to be especially suited to look after the bath. Alternatively, Fortuna, goddess of fate was often portrayed in bath-houses, in order to protect bathers when they were most vulnerable. In addition, there were countless nymphs and sprites associated with local springs and pools who were venerated as guardians of the bath.

■ Hydrotherapy – the bath in medicine

Although bathing was often recommended as a part of treatment throughout the centuries, it was not until the eighteenth century that it really came into its own.

Healing wells were used by people all over Europe from prehistoric times. The Celts and other races considered them sacred places and often erected shrines by them. When Christianity spread across the continent these healing wells and shrines were blessed and became incorporated into the Church as Holy wells.

In the sixteenth and seventeenth centuries many of these Holy wells became very important as various doctors began to extol the virtues of 'taking the waters.' Among these was Dr William Turner who published in 1562 *A booke of the nature and properties of the bathes of England* .. and other countries. Before long the era of the Spa towns had begun (all named after Spa in Belgium, the original centre). At these centres people would come to drink and/or bathe in the waters.

In the early nineteenth century Vincent Priessnitz (1799–1851), founded the method which was to be called Hydropathy (from hydro, meaning water and pathos, meaning suffering). Born in Grafenberg in Silesia (later to become known as Jesenic in Czechoslovakia), Priessnitz devised a method of treating people with a variety of baths and springs. No additives were made to the water and no claims were made for the minerals contained in it. The emphasis was entirely upon the use of cold water used upon the individual in baths, wraps, sprays, showers, sponges and rubs.

Priessnitz's reputation spread like wildfire and patients flocked from all over Europe. In the year 1839 alone, it is recorded that among his clientele he saw: twenty-two princes and princesses, one duke, one duchess, one hundred and forty-nine counts and countesses, eighty-eight barons and baronesses ... and many, many more of lesser rank!

Disciples of the Priessnitz method carried the practice of Hydropathy across the world. Two English physicians, Dr James Wilson and Dr James Gully, established a hydropathic centre in Malvern, England. Others followed suit and a succession of hydropathic hospitals and hotels were established throughout the British Isles.

■ The Turkish Bath

In the nineteenth century the Roman hot air bath was reintroduced to polite society. It had in fact been adopted earlier by the Turks, hence its name. The famous Victorian actress Lily Langtry, along with many others were keen to extol its virtues. In 1885 she is quoted as saying:

> *'I attribute my perfect health to the Turkish Bath which I take twice a week regularly. I find it keeps my skin in excellent condition, . . . and I think for small ailments the Turkish Bath is the best doctor to fly to.'*

■ Naturopathy – the Nature Cure

The middle and latter part of the nineteenth century saw the rise of the Nature Cure. A succession of practitioners followed Priessnitz, using bathing as part of their Nature Cures. In essence they were practising non-drug medicine, believing that one can stimulate the body to expel accumulated toxins using natural methods. When this is done the natural healing ability of the body will bring about a Nature Cure.

Johannes Schroth, an Austrian set up a clinic which emphasised dry diets. Pastor Sebastian Kneipp advocated hot and cold bath treatments. In America a number of conventionally trained doctors took the methods and refined them further. Dr Henry Lindlahr and Dr J.H. Kellog both practised Hydrotherapy and wrote extensively about the therapeutic value of water and the different types of bath.

Following their lead, Naturopathic Medicine has developed into a complete system of medicine which is practised throughout the world. One of the main methods of treatment is Hydrotherapy and the therapeutic use of different types of bathing.

■ Mud, Peat and Brine

Medical hydrology is the name that was given to the science of water for therapeutic purposes. This included its internal use, as it was taken at different spas according to its constituent gases and minerals, and its external use in the various types of baths which were employed.

Balneology, was a section within medical hydrology which referred to the use of the bath and the various types of substance which were added. Indeed, 'medicated baths' were used at various spas according to the qualities of the minerals in the surrounding areas. Salts, gases, mud, peat and fango (a type of clay) all came to be employed, all with specific indications.

Sea-bathing was a treatment which had been advocated by many physicians over the years. In 1750, Dr Richard Russel published his book *A Dissertation concerning the Use of Sea-water in Diseases of the Glands*. The effect of the book was to attract people away from the inland spa towns to the coastal spas where sea-bathing was available along with the benefits of the other hydropathic treatments. And this led to yet another specialisation of hydrotherapy. It was called *Thalassotherapy* – the use of brine, seawater and seaweeds in the treatment of illness.

■ Who uses Hydrotherapy today?

In the latter part of the twentieth century the use of hydrotherapy is regaining respectability as its benefits are again becoming clear. Very many people are well aware that they feel better when they take particular types of bath. They are also aware that some temperatures just do not suit them. And again, many therapists including Rheumatologists, General Practitioners, Sports

Medicine specialists, Physiotherapists, Naturopaths and Aromatherapists (and many others) are all finding that therapeutic and medicated baths offer ideal gentle means of easing pains and other ailments.

CHAPTER TWO

The Remedial Effects of Bathing

'Water, air and cleanliness are the chief articles in my pharmacopoeia'.
NAPOLEON BONAPARTE

There are three ways in which water and bathing can exert a remedial effect upon the body. Through the action of temperature on the skin, by the mechanical effects of water and rubbing, and by the subtle action of the additives in medicated baths.

■ The Skin and temperature

The skin is an extremely important organ in its own right. It is ninety per cent responsible for regulating the temperature of the body. It protects the inner tissues and organs from the outer environment and manufactures Vitamin D under the action of sunlight. But in addition it also has absorption and excretory functions. For this latter reason it is often called *the third kidney*.

The circulation to and within the skin takes up ten per cent of the blood volume of the body. Under the action of the autonomic nervous system the skin blood vessels – *the arterioles, capillaries and venules* – can be dilated or constricted. This effect can be profound, since it can markedly increase or decrease the amount of blood flowing through the skin. This obviously will affect the circulation to other deeper organs and structures.

When heat in any form is applied to the skin there is a reflex dilation of the skin blood vessels. This increased blood flow becomes obvious as reddening, flushing or blushing of the skin. This is afterwards followed by increased perspiration and loss of heat from the body. Conversely, when the skin is cooled there is a reflex constriction of the skin blood vessels. This decreased flow causes pallor, inhibition of perspiration and ultimately shivering.

As the temperature on the skin is increased there is a rise in the rate of flow of blood within the skin. This is accompanied by an increase in exchange of metabolic products between the blood and the skin tissue. Thus, oxygen and nutrients are quickly supplied to the skin cells and the metabolic waste products are removed.

■ The deeper effects of temperature

Whatever happens to the skin circulation automatically has an effect upon the internal organs. When external heat causes more blood to be diverted to the skin, the supply to the deeper tissues is reduced. The autonomic circulation brings in compensatory mechanisms to deal with this. This may result in temporary reduction in function. For example, the gastro-intestinal tract activity is reduced and the nervous system is sedated. In addition, the thyroid gland and adrenal glands seem to slow down. On the other hand, the heart rate increases to pump the blood to the skin. In addition, the breathing rate increases. This has the effect of blowing off carbon dioxide from the lungs, causing a very slight shift in the acid-base balance of the blood. If this lasts for some time, then the kidney starts to produce an alkaline urine to bring the acid-base balance back to normal.

Finally, moist heat, as from a bath, is extremely good for easing muscle spasm and the pain which often results from it.

When the skin is cooled, the opposite effects can be expected. The supply of blood to the deeper tissues and organs is increased. Since the body needs to maintain temperature, it does so by increasing metabolism. In part this may be because the thyroid produces more thyroxine, one of the main hormones which regulates the body's metabolic rate. In addition, the muscles are stimulated to produce heat by shivering. The appetite is also stimulated, in order to get more food or fuel into the body to stoke the fires of metabolism.

■ Perspiration

The main method by which the body loses its heat is through perspiration. If the body is immersed in water or wrapped so that the perspiration cannot evaporate, then this causes the heating effect upon the skin to become even more profound. When the perspiration is finally allowed to take place, after leaving the water, the excretory function of the skin comes into action. *The third kidney* will help to remove accumulated toxins.

This detoxification function of the skin is highly important in Hydrotherapy.

■ Temperature ranges

Different temperatures have different effects upon the body. In some circumstances a cold application will help, while at other times it will make matters worse. For this reason a whole range of temperatures are used in Hydrotherapy. For simplicity, however, we shall consider just three – cold, tepid and hot.

Cold – (50°–85°F; 10°–29°C), these temperatures are used to stimulate metabolism, diminish muscle irritability (after the shivering stops), tone up the skin, increase immunity. These temperatures should only be used by fit people with no heart or blood pressure problems. This is because the cold can produce an alteration in heart rate and a short rise in blood pressure.

The very lowest temperatures should only be used for a few seconds at a time. At the higher end of the range the maximum time should be two minutes.

Tepid – (85°–97°F; 29°–36°C), this range of temperature is similar to body temperature (98.4°F or 37°C), so we are not expecting profound physiological changes. There will not be much perspiration caused, so there will be little excretion of toxins. And there will not be stimulation of metabolism from the cold reaction.

The main remedial function of the tepid bath is to create a pleasant temperature for the individual to soak in a bath which has been medicated.

A tepid bath can be tolerated without undue problem for fifteen minutes to an hour.

Hot – (100°–107°F, 38°–41°C), this range is used when one wishes to stimulate the excretory role of the skin, to stimulate the 'third kidney' to aid detoxification.

This range is also very useful for the pain-killing effect the heat produces on muscles and joints. It is also beneficial for many problems associated with painful spasm-type pain.

Finally, the hot bath has a sedating and relaxing effect. For this reason it is best taken later in the day when one can lie down afterwards. It is beneficial in tension states and when troubled by insomnia.

They can be taken for between five and fifteen minutes, but should ideally be restricted to such times that the individual does not have to leave the house after them.

■ Mechanical effects upon the body

Archimedes' principle states that when a body is immersed in water it displaces its own weight in water.

Because the body is not so heavy in water, it is easier to move the limbs. Exercise in water is therefore excellent when there is restriction of movement from weakness or pain.

Water obviously washes the surface of the skin. This is useful when removing metabolic waste, but less desirable if it is reducing natural body oils. The individual should not bathe more than is necessary. For the well and fit person there is no need to bathe more than once a day. This is particularly important with hot baths, since they have an enhanced excretory potential. Quite simply, too many hot baths will deplete one's vitality and predispose to debility.

Counter-irritation of the skin also occurs if one has a painful condition. It is possible to stimulate fine nerve supplies in the skin in such a way that their stimulation will over-ride the painful impulses from the main pain condition. This may be one of the mechanisms of action of various showers, jacuzzis and douches. It may also explain the mode of action of some types (though not all) of medicated bath.

■ Medicated baths

The third means by which bathing can exert a remedial effect is through the use of additives to the bath. As mentioned above, some exert a counter-irritation effect. Others work by absorption of the substance through the skin. Here we include the use of things like seaweed, oatmeal and various herbal additives. Yet others work by the absorption of ingredients which have an altogether more subtle effect, as if they somehow directly affect the body's innate healing mechanisms. Here we include the various aromatherapy essential oils.

CHAPTER THREE

The Bath, Shower and Basin

A douche is a single or multiple column of water of varying temperature, pressure, and mass, directed against some portion of the body.

Dr J.H. KELLOG, 1918

The therapeutic armamentarium of Spa and Hydrotherapy practice includes a whole array of specialised baths, showers and basins. While some treatments can only really be given in specially converted hydropathic establishments, others are altogether simpler and can be used very satisfactorily in one's own bathroom. It is this latter group that we are concerned with.

■ Plain Baths

The standard European bath is a very versatile remedial tool. Used properly it can be used successfully in many conditions. To think of it as just a receptacle for washing water is to miss its true potential. If you use it in a methodical, thoughtful manner, rather than just in a 'pot-luck' way, then you will see how it can pep you up when your vitality is low or relax you when the going is tough.

Temperature – is important, as we considered in the last chapter. A thermometer is therefore an important addition to make to your bathroom cabinet. It should read in the range 50°–110°F: 10°–42°C. A clinical thermometer is likely to have too narrow a range, but a household one will do.

Remember, the temperature range, function and duration of the three types of bath are:-

1) Cold baths –
Range = (50°–85°F; 10°–29°C),
Function = Stimulation of metabolism
Duration = seconds to maximum of two minutes

2) Tepid baths –
Range = (85°–97°F; 29°–36°C),
Function = Comfortable medicated bathing
Duration = fifteen minutes to an hour

3) Hot –
Range = (100°–107°F, 38°–41°C),
Function = De-toxification through increased perspiration, relaxation, pain-relief
Duration = five to fifteen minutes

Depth – has to be considered, since it has a bearing upon the regulation of temperature and upon the posture the bather takes up in the bath. It also is of relevance in calculating how much of an additive to put in the bath.

In a standard European bath 2–2.5 gallons are needed per inch depth of water.

Posture – in a standard bath one can either sit up, lean on the back of the bath or lie with the main part of the body immersed. Obviously this will affect the amount of skin covered and the effect of temperature upon the skin.

A cold bath should ideally be a complete immersion of the body up to the neck for a short period. For most people this should only be done for literally a few seconds. A tepid bath can be taken in any posture, since it is mainly used as a medicated bath. Thus one can change the posture from sitting to lying. Obviously, if the medicated bath is being used for a general skin condition, then the parts of the skin affected should be covered for some of the time.

To get the maximum effect from a hot bath it should be of short duration, in a lying position, with the scalp dampened and possibly a cool cloth draped over the forehead.

Time – the length of time spent in the bath is important. A cold bath should be short and sharp and of no longer than a couple of minutes maximum. A tepid bath can be from fifteen minutes to an hour, although twenty minutes is long enough for remedial effect. Hot baths should like cold baths only be used for short duration, say a maximum of fifteen minutes for a warm-hot bath, or five minutes maximum for a very hot bath.

Cold reaction – to get the very best out of tepid and hot baths they should ideally be interspersed with a cold showering. That is, one should give oneself a swift showering of cold water during the bath. If the bath is not a combined bath and shower, then one of the rubber shower nozzles which can be attached to the taps is an effective compromise. Simply, once or twice during the bath sit up and take a very swift cool or cold shower over the upper trunk. After the last one, you get out and towel down briskly.

The effect of this is to produce a cold reaction. This effect, like the cold plunge in a swimming pool, slows the breathing and ultimately speeds up the metabolism.

IMPORTANT NOTE: EXTREMES OF TEMPERATURE HAVE POTENTIAL SIDE EFFECTS WHICH CAN BE UNDESIRABLE FOR CHILDREN, THE ELDERLY AND PEOPLE WITH CERTAIN CONDITIONS. PLEASE READ THE FOLLOWING CHAPTER ON DOs AND DON'Ts BEFORE EXPERIMENTING WITH BATHS.

■ Sitz Baths

As mentioned in Chapter One, the Ancient Greeks favoured Sitz baths. These are essentially hip baths, but with the feet in a separate receptacle containing water of a different temperature. Like plain baths, Sitz baths can be taken cold, tepid or hot, depending upon whether the aim is stimulation, medication or detoxification. In addition, they can be alternated in a Contrast Sitz bath.

Sitz baths are, as we shall see in the later chapters, particularly good for many types of abdominal and pelvic problem. They are, however, also very useful for people who are unable to take a plain immersion bath.

To make your own Sitz bath you need a large basin which can be fitted into the foot end of your main bath. A plastic baby bath is generally adequate, because it has sufficient depth. This is filled with cold water while the main bath is filled with the heated water. Once it is ready the individual sits upright in the main bath in about six inches of depth (enough to cover the hips and pelvis), with the feet in the cold basin.

Two minutes is the most you should stay in on the first occasion or two, gradually increasing the time to a maximum of ten minutes.

1) Hot Sitz bath – with the main bath in the hot temperature range, is useful for acute spasm pains in the abdomen and pelvis. It will have a tendency to induce perspiration and detoxification.

2) Tepid Sitz bath – with the main bath in the tepid temperature range, the main bath contains the medicated water. This is a relaxing Sitz bath which can be enjoyed for ten minutes. It is useful for less acute, but recurrent problems. It is used as a preventive and as a strengthener.

3) Cold Sitz bath – with the main bath in the cold range and the foot bath in the tepid or warm-hot range. This is used as a stimulant bath.

4) Contrast Sitz bath – this is taken as the hot Sitz bath, but only for two minutes. After that, one changes position to sit in the cold with the feet in the hot for another two minutes. This is repeated twice, in a total time of twelve minutes.

■ Medicated baths

These are baths to which something is added. Generally, warm-tepid and hot baths are used for this purpose. Cold baths are used so swiftly that there is not enough time for the additive to exert its effect.

Epsom Salt baths – these famous salts made from hydrated magnesium sulphate, named after the spa town of Epsom with its ancient healing salt spring, are extremely effective in easing pains of the musculo-skeletal system and in inducing a detoxification reaction.

To make the bath you take 500 grams of Epsom Salts (available from any chemist) and mix it with almond oil in a basin beside the bath to produce a pleasing wet sand feel.

Draw a hot-tepid bath, so that you will be able to get in with comfort. Stand in the bath and, taking a couple of handfuls of the mixture, rub it over yourself from the neck downwards. Use sweeping movements in the direction of the heart. Do not put on the face or around the genitals.

Put the rest of the Epsom Salt mixture into the bath and stir it with your hands. Then sit down and gently wash the salts off. Then lie down as you increase the temperature to a hot bath. Stay for up to ten minutes.

Having had the bath, shower down quickly with cold or lukewarm water. Take care not to get up too quickly or you might feel faint (See next chapter on Do's and Don'ts). Have a drink of fluid, then prepare for bed, making sure that you are wearing nightclothes. The perspiration reaction will take place during the night.

Take an Epsom salt bath every other day for a week to get a good detoxification reaction.

Sulphur baths – these used to be used for de-infesting people from lice. They were also used in Dermatology practice as a tepid bath. However, they have a great problem in that they can easily produce an eczematous reaction in a fair proportion of people. For that reason I mention them out of interest only.

Oatmeal baths – these are extremely good for the skin. Take 500 grams of oatmeal and tie in a large muslin cloth. This should be hung over the side of the bath under the hot tap, so that the running water flows through the bundle. This should be a tepid bath. You get in and relax the whole body in the bath for as long as you like. Twenty minutes to half an hour should be sufficient therapeutically.

Alternatively, you can soak the oatmeal overnight in a bucket containing a gallon of water. This you mix directly into the bath which you run up to tepid temperature.

These baths can be repeated as often as necessary.

Mud, Peat and Clay baths – these have been used at different spas for centuries. Indeed, the Ancient Greeks advocated the bathing in the mud from certain areas, believing them to be full of healing potential.

The benefits of *peloid*, as mud and peat additives are referred to therapeutically, are said to arise from the organic compounds and minerals which have accumulated over the years. The properties are said to vary according to the minerals and plants found in the area the peloid was obtained from.

Partly, they work by causing some absorption of the compounds through the skin. And partly they work by inducing a detoxification reaction.

Mud from Neydharting in Austria is said to contain natural antibiotics, large quantities of vitamins, minerals and trace elements. Packs of this mud extract are available from many health shops.

Mud baths are given in hydropathic hotels and health farms for rheumatism, chronic skin problems, various gynaecological disorders and for general toning up. They can either be taken as full mud baths or as wraps. Wraps seem to be the most sensible type to use at home.

Peat baths can be taken at home using liquid peat extract, rather than peat. Again, the best seem to be those of Austrian origin. These also can be obtained from health shops. Simply use a hot-tepid bath and add the recommended quantity. Soak in this for up to fifteen minutes. This should be done last thing at night, like an Epsom Salt bath, after which one should drink some fluid and retire to bed. A perspiration reaction will take place during the night.

Clay baths are also useful, because they induce a powerful detoxification reaction. They do this because they actually seem to draw toxins out through the skin.

French Green Clay, called *Bentonite*, can be bought from many health shops. A hot-tepid bath should be drawn and 500 grams of the French Green Clay should be added and stirred to dissolve. One reclines completely in the bath for up to ten minutes, topping up with hot water to create a hot bath for a maximum of five more minutes.

As with an Epsom Salt bath, one should shower off any surplus with cold or lukewarm water before drying off, drinking a little fluid and retiring to bed. A perspiration reaction can be expected in the night.

Seaweed baths – a complete branch of hydrotherapy is called Thalassotherapy. The name comes from the group of Thallophyta, to which seaweed belongs. It actually utilises both seawater and seaweed. The seawater, or brine is used to enhance the buoyancy of the water, thereby allowing the body to be partially supported during exercise.

The seaweed is used in the same way as peat. That is, for the organic compounds, vitamins and minerals that can be absorbed through the skin, and for its effect in inducing perspiration and detoxification. Great care has to be taken, however, if the individual is allergic to iodine (see next chapter on Do's and Don'ts).

Salt baths can easily be taken at home without the necessity of obtaining seawater! They can be taken like the Epsom Salt bath. They are good for detoxification and perspiration induction. They are also very good for genital and various types of skin and chronic infections.

Begin by drawing a hot-tepid bath, so that you will be able to get in with comfort. In a basin by the bath dissolve 500 grams of common salt in just enough water to turn it into a paste. Take a handful or two of the paste and slowly rub the mixture over the body from the neck downwards. Use sweeping circular movements in the direction of the heart. Do not put on the face or around the genitals. Having done that, put the rest of the mixture into the bath and stir it with your hands. Then sit down and gently wash the salt off. Then lie down as you increase the temperature to a hot bath. Stay for up to ten minutes.

Having had the bath, shower down quickly with cold or lukewarm water. Take care not to get up too quickly or you might feel faint (See

32

next chapter on Do's and Don'ts). Have a drink of fluid, then prepare for bed, making sure that you are wearing nightclothes. The perspiration reaction will take place during the night.

Herbal baths – these have many excellent indications, as you will see in the following chapters. The basic method of using them is with a tepid bath in which one can soak. Generally speaking fifteen to twenty minutes is enough for therapeutic purposes, but one can happily stay in for up to an hour.

Use 50–100 grams of the dried herb in a muslin cloth and hang it under the hot running tap. Then hang it into the water and allow it to infuse. This can either be used in a plain or a Sitz bath.

Alternatively, one can make up an infusion or decoction of the herb in a gallon of water, which is then added to the bath. Tepid water is added to the right temperature.

An *infusion* is prepared by adding the herb to boiled water and leaving, as one does when making tea. This is the favoured way for soft, fleshy herbs. A *decoction* is made by adding the herb to water which is then boiled and simmered for about quarter of an hour, then left to infuse for another six hours. This is better when using woody herbs.

Yet another method which might appeal is to use herbal tea bags. You will find that most health shops stock many herbal teas in tea-bag cartons. Four or five tea bags can be used in a quick herbal bath.

Aromatherapy baths – again, these are taken as tepid baths. Simply, 6–8 drops of the chosen essential oil are added to the bath. One soaks in it for fifteen to twenty minutes.

■ Aerated baths

Some people have spas or jacuzzis in their home. These are the equivalent of the old-fashioned aerated bath. Their effectiveness is mainly from the mechanical effect of the streams of bubbles which hit the skin. They are stimulating.

Effervescent baths – these are plain baths to which a special foaming agent, such as the once famous and much prescribed *Balneum Effervescens cum Chloridis (BPC)*, is added. The foaming which takes place at a tepid temperature, is again thought to stimulate the skin and muscles and produce a pleasing relaxing effect.

■ Saunas

These have always been popular in Scandinavia and have started to become popular in Britain, especially in health clubs. Some people even have saunas built in their own homes.

Saunas can either be taken as whole body treatments or as partial treatments. The latter method is well-suited and convenient for the home.

Saunas depend upon the promotion of a perspiration and detoxification reaction. The heat stimulates the circulation of the skin and helps establish a relaxation response. The moistness or humidity inhibits perspiration initially (because it does not allow adequate evaporation) and therefore causes the internal heat to rise. When one is removed from the heat, the perspiration reaction continues.

Partial saunas – this is the old fashioned bowl of boiled water and towel approach. It is extremely beneficial to the skin. Simply, add the appropriate herb or aromatherapy oil to a bowl of steaming water and lean over it with a towel over your head to form a simple sauna tent. This will open the skin pores and allow local detoxification to take place.

■ Showers and Douches

Hydrotherapy lays a lot of emphasis upon the use of showers. A whole range of different types of shower are used in hydropathic establishments, just as they were once used in rheumatological hospitals.

Cold showers are very stimulating – hence their advocated use in spartan training establishments throughout the world. Hot showers, on the other hand, will induce a perspiration reaction, so they should not be taken for too long (five or ten minutes maximum, remembering that they may be at a higher temperature than one could tolerate a hot bath) and they are always best finished with a cold wash down to close the skin pores. They are best taken at the end of the day.

Showers cannot be properly medicated, and it is not advisable to use the salt or Epsom salt treatment with a shower, because of the very real risk of dropping blood pressure and inducing a faint.

The real benefit of showers is in their mechanical role. Here one has to consider the power of the jets and the area which they are directed at. When used therapeutically, one ideally wishes to be able to vary both of these.

Regarding pressure, quite simply, the faster the water comes out, the more stimulating the effect upon the skin.

Regarding the area treated, the broader the area covered by the spray, the less the local stimulation. Conversely, the narrower the spray, the greater the stimulation to the skin.

Overhead showers – domestic showers can either be static or moveable. The moveable one is the most useful, since one can use it to direct the spray at local areas of the body. This obviously means that one would be able to vary the pressure of the flow hitting the skin.

Bath showers – many domestic showers are combined with the bath. Some directly divert water from the bath taps, while others have an independent supply going up through a heating box. A bath shower is excellent for showering off after various types of bath.

Other types of douche – this refers to the use of water or solutions directed into a body cavity, in order to irrigate, cleanse or disinfect.

Nasal douches – these are often of use in respiratory problems and when there is a problem with recurrent infections elsewhere in the body (because sometimes one can carry the infecting organism in the nose). An infusion of the appropriate solution is drawn up in a dropper (of the type which can be purchased from chemists complete with a 30ml bottle for keeping the fluid). With the head over the bath or hand basin, and with the head on the side so that the nostril to be treated is uppermost, a dropperful is instilled into the nostril while the other is kept closed. Wait for as long as you can (twenty seconds is a good time), then turn your head and allow the fluid to drain out. Repeat with the other nostril.

Nasal douches are not to be used with toddlers (see next chapter on Dos and Don'ts).

Vaginal douches – these can be obtained from chemists and many health shops. They are for gentle instillation of fluid into the vagina. They are of value with recurrent or persistent vaginal irritation or discharge. Obviously, they must be kept scrupulously clean. They usually come complete with a bulb chamber or bag and special vaginal tubing. Usually a special valve is included so that the pressure generated will not be to great. The idea is to use it while in the bath. The chamber is filled and the tubing inserted into the entrance to the vagina. The bulb variety is worked like a syringe, while the bag variety is operated by gravity. In the latter type the chamber is raised so that the fluid is gently instilled into the vagina. A slight feeling of fullness may be felt. The chamber is lowered and the tubing removed, allowing the fluid to gradually flow out.

Rectal douches or enemas – these too are advocated by many naturopaths to relieve toxins from the body. However, where there is an alteration of bowel habit or a tendency to chronic constipation, it is sensible to seek professional help rather than attempt to manage the problem alone. (Please see the next chapter about Dos and Don'ts).

At the time of writing this book it is possible to get a bulb chamber syringe complete with either rectal or vaginal tubing, for enema or douche, on presentation of a doctor's prescription.

■ Basins

Here we refer to basins and buckets which can easily be adapted for use in the bathroom. They are used when we wish to apply a local treatment to a part of the body. We have already considered the use of the basin in a facial sauna and for inhalations. Others include:-

Foot baths – here a basin or bucket is needed which can be placed on the floor. It can be used for either hot or cold water, either with or without medication. It should be deep enough to cover as far up the lower leg as possible. To the knee is ideal, but if this is not possible then at least a couple of inches above the ankles.

Mustard foot bath – this is a particular type of foot bath. It is used with hot water. A heaped tablespoonful of mustard powder is added to the basin or bucket of hot water.

Hand and arm baths – these are exactly the same as the foot baths. They are very useful for many arthritic and rheumatic problems.

■ Wraps, Compresses and Gloves

These are occlusive methods of treatment which are either used to produce an intense detoxification reaction, or to enhance the effect of a medication to a local area.

Body wrap – these are used to create an intense detoxification reaction through the skin. They do so by producing heat and promoting perspiration.

A cotton sheet is taken and dampened with cold water. It should not be soaking. It is placed on top of a blanket. The individual lies on this and then wraps the sheet round the body. A couple of hot water bottles are then insinuated between the sheet and the blanket (one at the feet and one at the waist). The blanket is wrapped around the body.

A perspiration reaction takes place within ten minutes. The individual usually falls asleep soon after. The wrap should be left for three hours. When it is unwrapped the sheet will be bone dry, but may be stained. The individual should then sponge clean.

THIS IS ONLY TO BE DONE BY THE VERY FIT AND WELL. IT IS ABSOLUTELY CONTRA-INDICATED FOR ANYONE WITH HIGH BLOOD PRESSURE OR A HEART PROBLEM.

Partial body wraps – these are mini-versions of the whole body wrap. They can be used to generate heat in the part concerned – the limbs or the trunk.

Compresses – these are useful methods of reducing localised areas of inflammation. A cloth or towel is folded so that it will fit or mould to the area of the body concerned. It is soaked in hot or cold water as appropriate, then wrung out. A hot compress should not be so hot that it cannot be comfortably held against the skin. It is held in place until it cools.

A cold compress is held or bound to the area and left until it is no longer cold. It can be left overnight if necessary.

Alternating hot and cold compresses can be used for acute traumas and inflammations. The hot compress is left for three minutes, then replaced by the cold compress for a minute. This cycle is repeated for up to about twenty minutes.

Gloves – washing-up gloves are excellent for giving heat treatment to the hands and wrists. A basin is filled with hot water (comfortable) as the gloves are put on. They are then rested in the water, but without the water being allowed into the glove.

This is also good for occlusion methods of treatment using aromatherapy oils or herbal ointments. The ointment is applied to the hands and wrists, then the gloves are slipped on. Then the hands are rested in the hot water as above.

One can also improvise the same sort of occlusive treatment for the feet and ankles with plastic bags. The temperature should be warm-hot, rather than hot.

■ Friction Rubs

Actual stimulation of the skin by friction helps to tone up this highly important organ. The simplest thing to use is a loofah or natural fine bristle brush. This is done while the skin is dry. Starting at the soles of the feet brush or sweep with long movements in the direction of the heart. Work up the body, avoiding genitalia and nipples and face, always remembering to work in the direction of the heart. This is an excellent technique to absorb into your regular daily routine.

Salt glow – common salt is another excellent agent which can be used in a friction rub. It is taken in a similar way to the Epsom Salt bath. About 500 grams of salt should be mixed with enough water to make a sludge. Then sitting in the empty bath take a handful of salt and rub it over the feet and up the legs, using long vigorous sweeps. Do the limbs then the back, then the front of the trunk. As with the dry friction rub, always rub in the direction of the heart, and do not treat genitalia, nipples or face and neck.

Then wash the salt off with your hand-shower or a quick warm bath. After that dry down briskly and go to bed. A perspiration reaction and sleepiness are liable to follow.

CHAPTER FOUR

Do's and Don'ts

Whatever was required to be done, the Circumlocution Office was beforehand with all the public departments in the art of perceiving – HOW NOT TO DO IT.
CHARLES DICKENS, *Little Dorrit*

While most of the bathroom remedies in this book are beneficial, there are a few do's and don'ts that you should be aware of.

■ Do's

● Be sure what type of bath you are having – hot bath, Sitz bath, medicated bath, etc.

● Do make sure that you can get into the bath safely.

● Do make sure that you can comfortably tolerate the bath temperature. Do not run a hot bath and get straight in. Run a warm bath, get in then increase the temperature by adding hot water. Similarly, take care with a cold bath.

● Do use a thermometer to keep the temperature of the bath within the limits suggested in Chapter 3.

● Do restrict the time taken in the bath to the suggested times in Chapter 3.

● Do follow the maker's recommendations to the letter when using vaginal or other types of douche.

■ Don'ts

● Do not have a lock on the bathroom door, unless absolutely essential.

● Do not take alcohol or powerful drugs before a bath.

● Do not take a bath after a heavy meal. Two hours should be the minimum, but preferably three hours.

● Do not take a hot bath or a hot Sitz bath if there is a history of high blood pressure or heart disease. Have a medical check first.

● Do not use a Salt glow or take an Epsom Salt bath if there is a history of high blood pressure or heart disease. Have a medical check first.

● Do not take hot baths, hot Sitz baths, Salt glow or Epsom Salt baths if pregnant.

● Do not take aromatherapy baths when pregnant, unless for a few specific conditions (see Chapter 9).

● Do not submit children to hot baths, hot Sitz baths, Epsom Salt baths or Salt glows.

● Do not get up too quickly after an Epsom Salt bath, a Salt bath, a wrap, or a hot bath. There may be a drop in blood pressure causing unwanted dizziness or even fainting.

● Do not use Bladderwrack (seaweed) in a bath if there is a history of allergy to iodine.

● Do not use additives in a bath if there is a strong history of skin allergy. It is quite safe to test a solution on a part of the body (eg the thigh) before taking such a bath.

● Do not stay longer than the recommended times, particularly with hot baths and detoxification remedies.

- Do not take hot baths if feeling debilitated or low in energy. They will debilitate you more.

- Do not take a hot bath or shower without cool showering down or cooling with cold water. This is necessary to close down the pores.

- Do not take hot baths too early in the day if you have to go out again.

- Do not take cold baths if suffering from intercurrent infections of the respiratory tract.

- Do not take hot baths if there is any neurological impairment of sensation.

- Do not take hot baths if there is any peripheral vascular problem, such as intermittent claudication. This is manifested by pain in the calf muscles on walking short distances.

- Do not take hot baths if there are any vascular complications of Diabetes Mellitis, such as leg ulceration.

- Do not administer nasal douches or internal douches of any sort to children.

■ Help for the disabled

Bathing is something which most able-bodied people take for granted. For many disabled and elderly people this is not feasible. Yet many of the bathroom remedies can still benefit them, albeit taken in modified form.

If someone has restricted mobility and cannot lie down in the bath, or even sit down, then a bath stool or bath seat may be useful. Bath rails may also help, either fitted to the side of the bath or the front of the bath at the taps end.

Usually an Occupational Therapist can be asked to visit, after referral by the family doctor. They are highly skilled in assessing the needs of people with physical weakness or sensory problems. They can then make recommendations for appropriate fitments to be installed.

The disabled are advised to avoid the extreme temperature therapeutic baths and restrict bathing to medicated baths. If the individual is restricted to a bath seat, high above the water level, then the medicated bath can still be used as outlined in the book. Indeed, if the individual cannot use a bath seat or stool, then a medicated foot bath with a medicated hand basin will still suffice.

The herbal medicated foot and hand baths are still made in the same proportions. If the chosen herb is available as a 'tea-bag' then this is a simple way of usage. One or two of the herbal tea-bags are tossed into the foot bath and hand basin and allowed to infuse.

The aromatherapy medicated foot and hand baths are made with half the quantity of essential oils added – 3 or 4 drops will be quite sufficient.

A medicated herbal or aromatherapy partial bath (as just described) can be finished off by soaking a towel in the solution and having a wrap around the trunk for up to five minutes. The solution should only be applied warm and should not be left until it is cold.

Sitz baths can be improvised in a shower, by sitting on a safe stool in the shower, with the feet in a basin of medicated cold solution, while a warm shower is sprayed over the lower back. This can then be reversed, by replacing the basin with warm-hot water and spraying cool water over the trunk. Obviously, however, a disabled person should not attempt such a procedure without an able-bodied person around to help or offer support.

SECTION TWO

THE REMEDIES

CHAPTER FIVE

Arthritis, Rheumatism & Sprains

Pain and stiffness from musculo-skeletal problems are among the commonest of all health complaints. Indeed, it is one of the areas where hydrotherapy of some form can definitely help.

■ Aching feet and legs

This symptom can have many different causes. It can reflect metabolic problems or a problem with the circulation. If it is persistent then a medical opinion should be sought.

Mustard foot baths – are excellent for aching feet and calf pains. The feet are placed in and rested in the foot bath for about fifteen minutes, then toweled dry.

Medicated herbal baths – Arnica or Sage in a warm bath work very well with most muscular types of leg aching.

Medicated aromatherapy baths – Add 6–8 drops of Cypress, Eucalyptus, Marjoram, Pine or Sage essential oils to a warm bath.

■ Acute sprains and strains

Always ensure that there are no broken bones. Having had that excluded, one can ease many soft tissue injuries and ease swelling and inflammation with appropriate hydrotherapy treatment.

Alternating hot and cold compresses – can be used for acute traumas and inflammations. The hot compress is left for three minutes, then replaced by the cold compress for a minute. This cycle is repeated for up to about twenty minutes.

Herbal limb baths – these are very useful for many sports injuries where there is no break in the skin. These are used after the first aid treatment with alternating compresses has reduced the acute inflammation.

Tendonitis, Tennis Elbow, Golfer's Elbow, tenosynovitis and local sprains are among the conditions amenable to such treatment.

Arnica, Comfrey, Sage and Witch Hazel are all very useful. A pint is infused and placed in a limb bath containing about a gallon of warm, comfortable water. The limb is rested in this for fifteen minutes. This can be repeated three or four times a day.

Aromatherapy limb baths – Add 3–4 drops of Eucalyptus, Lavender or Marjoram essential oils to a warm limb bath. Alternatively, add 6–8 drops to a full bath.

■ General muscular strains

Here we mean the general aches and pains which come about through more exertion than one is used to. A vigorous game of squash after a long lay-off, a heavy day in the garden, that sort of general aching. Often you perform the activity and think that you have gotten away with it, only to be smitten the next day. It is best to take precautions by treating it prophylactically on the day of the exertion.

Hot bath – a hot bath taken in the range of 100°–107°F (38°–41°C), for a mere five minutes will ease pains if they are being experienced acutely. One should shower down with tepid water then get out, dry down and wrap up well. You do not want to induce a full perspiration reaction.

Medicated herbal bath – Arnica or Sage in a warm bath work very well with most general muscular aches.

Medicated aromatherapy bath – Add 6–8 drops of Cypress, Eucalyptus, Marjoram or Sage essential oils to a warm bath.

■ Osteoarthritis

This is the general 'wear and tear' type of arthritis. It commonly begins in the thirties, affecting joints which have been 'overused.' All joints can be affected, especially the spine, knees, hips and hands. By the age of 65 years 80–90 per cent of the population have X-ray evidence of Arthritis, although only about 20 per cent have pain from it.

Medicated herbal baths – Bladderwrack (seaweed), Comfrey and Nettle all individually work well in a warm bath with many cases of Osteoarthritis.

Medicated aromatherapy baths – Add 6–8 drops of Benzoin, Cedarwood, Chamomile or Lavender to a warm bath.

Medicated Sitz baths – these are particularly good for treating lower limb Osteoarthritis. All of the above herbs or oils can be used in the warm bath.

Medicated gloves – (see chapter 3) This is a good way of treating local Arthritis of the hand and wrist. Smear Comfrey ointment over the affected parts then slip on a pair of rubber washing-up gloves. Then rest the gloved hands in a warm basin for up to fifteen minutes. This can be repeated a couple of times a day when they are particularly troublesome.

■ Gout

This painful condition is caused by the accumulation of uric acid crystals in joints, classically the big toe, but also the knee. Diuretic tablets can provoke an attack.

Medicated herbal baths – Celery or Nettle in a warm bath often work very well with gout.

Medicated aromatherapy baths – Add 6–8 drops of Rosemary or Thyme to a bath. They can alternatively be placed in a foot bath if the toe is mainly affected.

Medicated sock – (see Chapter 3) This is a variant of the medicated glove. Comfrey ointment smeared over the affected joint is then covered by placing the foot in a plastic bag. This is then immersed in a lukewarm foot bath for up to fifteen minutes.

■ Sciatica

This is a pain caused by stimulation of the sciatic nerve. There are many possible causes so a medical opinion is necessary. It produces pain radiating from the back, through the buttock all the way down to the foot.

Medicated Sitz bath – this is an excellent method of treating sciatica, provided that the individual has sufficient mobility to adopt the posture needed by a Sitz bath.

A herbal Sitz bath with Basil, Thyme and Nettle all seem to work well to help soothe the discomfort of this condition.

An aromatherapy Sitz bath made by adding 6–8 drops of Eucalyptus, Chamomile or Lavendar essential oils may help.

■ Infammatory Arthritis

There are many types of Arthritis which are caused by an auto-immune Inflammatory

Arthritis. The most important of these is Rheumatoid Arthritis, but conditions like Ankylosing Spondylosis, Ulcerative Colitis and Psoriasis also produce a similar problem.

Medicated gloves and socks – as for Osteoarthritis often work well if there is small joint involvement.

Hot baths – a hot bath taken in the range of 100°–107°F (38°–41°C), for about ten minutes, followed by cold showering off will induce a perspiration reaction. This done last thing at night on three nights a week will often help mild to moderate cases by inducing detoxification.

Epsom Salt bath – an Epsom Salt bath every other day for a week will also produce a good detoxification reaction. This can be extremely helpful. (see Chapter 4 on Dos and Don'ts).

The Salt glow and Dry Friction rubs – both of these are worth doing regularly. A Salt Glow once a week will often help to keep the excretory and detoxifying function of the skin at optimum levels. A Dry rub should be part of the Inflammatory Arthritis individual's daily routine.

Medicated herbal baths – Celery and Nettle seem to help some cases of mild to moderate Inflammatory Arthritis.

Medicated aromatherapy bath – Add 6–8 drops of Juniper essential oil. This is extremely good for Rheumatoid Arthritis.

CHAPTER SIX

Skin Problems

Many people take their skin for granted. It is in fact an extremely important organ which protects our delicate inner structures from the hostile environment, manufactures Vitamin D from the sun, and acts in a number of ways to maintain the internal status quo. And as covered in Chapter 2, it also has very important absorption and excretion functions.

Finally, the way we feel is often reflected in the way our skin looks. Truly, the skin is the mirror of the mind.

For most skin conditions:-

1) The depth of the water should be waist deep. That is reaching to the tummy button while sitting in the bath.

2) The temperature of the water should be tepid-warm — 85°–97°F (29°–36°C), preferably nearer the bottom of the range. You do not want the temperature to be too hot, since this merely increases irritation. Indeed, many skin conditions are exacerbated by being too hot.

■ Eczema

Eczema or Dermatitis refers to inflammation of the skin. It is due to a general allergic reaction of the body, or it is due to local inflammation through direct contact with something which one is allergic to. Atopic individuals often have alternating episodes of Asthma and Eczema.

In Contact Dermatitis there is a local reaction which is usually obvious. Common sensitisers are soap powders, metal jewellery or metal clothes fasteners.

Peat baths – a medicated bath in the temperature range of 85°–97°F (29°–36°C), to which liquid peat extract has been added is beneficial to this skin problem because of the cooling nature of the peat and its alkalinity. This latter effect helps to neutralise some of the acidic toxins accumulating upon the inflamed skin. After soaking in the bath for up to twenty minutes, shower off any residues, dab towel dry then retire to bed. One can expect to perspire during the night as the skin responds. Such a bath once or twice a week may help to settle the problem considerably during a flare-up.

Alkaline bath – a simple first aid soothing bath can be made when the skin is hot and intensely itchy. Add 75–100 grams (about 3–4 ounces) of bicarbonate of soda to a waist deep bath. This will soothe most intense itchy conditions.

Oatmeal baths – are traditional, but excellent treatments for Eczema. They are also excellent for soothing the skin if it is irritated after using a Salt Glow or taking an Epsom Salt bath.

Medicated herbal baths – Elecampane, Chamomile and Lavender herbal baths are all very soothing to inflamed eczematous skin. Urtica, or the Common Nettle is also very useful for soothing raw inflamed Eczema.

Medicated aromatherapy baths – Bergamot, Chamomile, Juniper, Lavender, Myrrh and Rosemary are all good choices for Eczema.

■ Psoriasis

This condition is characterised by raised, scaly, silvery lesions, typically occurring in well-circumscribed lesions with a tendency to clear centrally.

The above peat, alkaline and oatmeal baths can all help.

Salt bath – a Salt bath taken as in Chapter 3, without the Salt rub over actual lesions, twice a week may help to stimulate the skin into a recovery pattern.

Medicated herbal baths – Urtica or Common Nettle baths are very good at helping the scaling lesions to heal.

Medicated aromatherapy baths – Bergamot, Lavender and Tea-tree oil are all beneficial in Psoriasis.

■ Sunburn, intense itch and acutely inflamed skin

All of these conditions are very uncomfortable, and need cooling. A tepid bath should be drawn with either an infusion of Urtica or Common Nettle (herbal bath) or 6–8 drops of one of the following – Clary Sage, Lavender, Geranium, Myrrh, Peppermint or Rose oils (aromatherapy bath).

■ Acne

This is one of the most embarrassing conditions for teenagers. It is characterised by a range of lesions all of which arise from the sebaceous activity of the skin. There can be whiteheads, blackheads, pustules and post-lesional scarring.

Partial saunas – the method for this is described in chapter 3. I have found that a herbal partial sauna using grated nutmeg (one pinch or small teaspoon per bowl of hot water) works well at stimulating detoxification in facial acne. The treatment will often cause a flaring up of the condition for a few days, followed by 'normal-isation' of the skin.

Medicated herbal baths – body acne will often also respond to a medicated herbal bath containing a decoction of horseradish (see Chapter 3).

Medicated aromatherapy baths – with either Bergamot, Chamomile, Sandalwood or Tea-tree oils is also very beneficial.

■ Varicose veins and aching legs

This condition can be really troublesome for many people. Varicosities are caused by back pressure upon the valves within the veins. Some people are fortunate and have more valves in their veins, so they never develop the problem. Once Varicose Veins have developed one cannot cure them (except with surgery), but there are several things which can be done to help.

Medicated herbal baths – Sage in the bath is an excellent remedy for easing the discomfort of varicose veins.

A Sage bath is also an excellent restorative for aching muscles and joints. This can be combined with heating a handful of salt then sprinkling it over a dry flannel. Wrap the flannel about the legs and leave on for about ten to fifteen minutes. It can be repeated if necessary. Alternatively, one can use the Salt glow (If the constitution will tolerate it), as outlined in Chapter 3.

IMPORTANT NOTE – The salt treatment must not be done if the skin is weak, broken, or prone to ulceration.

Mustard foot bath – this is an old and favoured remedy for aching feet and legs.

Medicated aromatherapy baths – Cypress and Lemon oils added to a bath are good for soothing Varicose Veins.

■ Chilblains

These are intensely itching and often painful conditions caused by damp cold to the extremities.

Medicated herbal foot baths – three Snowdrop bulbs chopped and crushed, then infused in a pint of hot water make an excellent preparation for a foot bath. This must be taken at a tepid temperature, since excess heat will provoke the chilblains. A couple of tablespoons to a simple nightly tepid footbath will often improve the condition swiftly.

Medicated aromatherapy baths – Lemon oil in a tepid bath is often effective.

■ Hair

Dandruff will often respond to a regular hair rinse with a Nettle or Rosemary herbal infusion. The simplest way of doing this is by using the appropriate tea-bags.

Soaking in an aromatherapy bath with either Chamomile, Lavender or Rosemary oils is also said to help the hair, if the scalp is rinsed occasionally with the water.

CHAPTER SEVEN

Chest and Breathing Problems

We have seen a change in chest conditions over the past two decades. While Tuberculosis has well nigh gone, and Chronic Bronchitis and Emphysema are less common, we see more and more cases of Acute Bronchitis and Asthma. Medical treatment is essential for these problems, but supportive treatment can make a substantial contribution to general well-being.

■ Coughs, colds and catarrh

No-one can ever entirely escape from the common cold. There are no mystical cures, but the following may help.

Gargles – Sage gargles can often ease a sore throat. Some people often find that a Salt Water gargle will also help.

Partial sauna – Eucalyptus oil, Lavender, Sandalwood or Tea-tree oils (3–4 drops in a bowl of hot water with a towel as a canopy can ease the upper respiratory congestion of an upper respiratory infection).

Sinusitis will often respond to a partial sauna with Cajeput, Eucalyptus, Lavender, or Tea-tree oil.

Compresses – alternating a hot with a cold compress to the forehead, cheeks and base of the skull, for up to five minutes at a time for twenty minutes will help to ease the pains of Sinusitis.

Cold Sitz baths – Chronic Catarrh will often respond to a daily cold Sitz bath for up to five minutes at a time, for a week.

Mustard foot baths – taken every night during a cold (see Chapter 3) may ease the aching feelings one experiences with a feverish cold.

Medicated herbal baths – Elecampane and Hyssop are both useful additions to a warm medicated bath every other evening during the cold.

Medicated aromatherapy baths – Benzoin, Black Pepper, Eucalyptus, Lavender, Sandalwood or Tea-Tree oil to a warm bath in the evenings will often loosen the congestion, soothe the cough and make you feel more comfortable.

■ Hay Fever

The problem here is allergy to grass or tree pollens. This needs to be tackled with conventional antihistamines or homoeopathic remedies. In addition, a cold plunge of the face in a basin every morning and evening, together with a daily cold Sitz bath, can bring relief.

■ Asthma

The diagnosis of many chest problems has become blurred over the last few years as it has become apparent that many conditions have a reversible degree of airway spasm. Medical treatment has improved, but it also has to be observed that the number of Asthma sufferers has increased dramatically.

Medical treatment should be continued at all costs, but the following measures may be helpful.

Medicated herbal baths – Basil, Elecampane, Eucalyptus, Lavender and Thyme in a warm medicated bath for twenty minutes at a time on a regular basis twice a week can help to maintain good breathing.

Medicated aromatherapy bath – Benzoin, Cajeput, Cypress, Frankincense, Lavender, Myrrh, Rosemary or Thyme are all potentially very helpful.

■ Chronic Bronchitis and Emphysema

These conditions can be helped by medicated baths. The steam produced acts as a mucolytic (catarrh-breaker) so the bath should be warm-hot.

Medicated herbal bath – a regular Elecampane bath taken twice or three times a week will often soothe the chronic catarrh and cough of these conditions.

Medicated aromatherapy bath – Cedarwood, Eucalyptus and Frankincense oils in a warm bath taken two or three times a week will often help the breathing of the individual.

HEART PROBLEMS

People who have had a heart attack, or who suffer from irregularly beating hearts or angina should not have baths which are too hot. They should always restrict the temperature of their bath to the temperature range of 85°–97°F; 29°–36°C. Above this they will induce a perspiration reaction which has a significant effect in diverting blood to the peripheries. This could easily provoke an attack of angina in someone with an impaired cardiovascular system.

■ Palpitations

This is the name for a symptom which has many potential causes. It is an awareness of the beating of the heart. Every case should be reported to your health adviser.

Medicated aromatherapy baths1 – Ylang Ylang oil is often very effective at reducing the speed of a fast heart rate.

Lavender, Rose and Rosemary are all very good at reducing the frequency of heavy beating, episodic thumping and irregular beating.

■ Angina

This is the name given to painful (usually left sided) chest pain occurring on exertion and relieved by rest. It too, should always be reported to and treated by your health adviser.

Medicated aromatherapy baths – Rosemary and Ylang Ylang oils may exert a soothing effect in angina.

■ High Blood Pressure

This is included here for convenience only. High blood pressure is generally divided into essential hypertension, accounting for 95–97 per cent of cases, and secondary hypertension, accounting for the remainder. The former is a direct problem related to the circulation. The latter group refers to a number of causes, including hormonal, kidney and systemic disorders.

Medicated aromatherapy bath – Chamomile, Lavender, Ylang Ylang oils are all effective in helping to control high blood pressure.

CHAPTER EIGHT

Abdominal Problems

Here we are mainly concerned with disorders of the gastro-intestinal tract and of the urinary system.

■ Heartburn

This symptom means the sensation of burning in the chest, often coming after a meal 'which disagrees', or after bending down. It is the result of acid from the stomach being spurted back into the oesophagus. Since the acid produces inflammation in the oesophagus the individual feels a burning pain.

The main treatment is with compounds which neutralise the acidity, or which prevent the spurting back of the acid. In addition, the following types of bath can help.

Medicated herbal bath – Fennel or Chamomile in a warm medicated bath for twenty minutes twice or three times a week.

Medicated aromatherapy bath – Black Pepper or Lemon oils in a warm bath for twenty minutes twice or three times a week.

■ Nausea and appetite stimulation

For a sickly feeling of gastro-intestinal origin the following can help.

Medicated herbal bath – Fennel, Chamomile or Peppermint infusions are all quite good at easing Nausea and helping to stimulate the appetite.

Medicated aromatherapy oils – Black Pepper, Chamomile, Ginger, Peppermint and Thyme are all helpful in this instance.

■ Gall Bladder problems

These classically affect women in their forties who have had children. Upper abdominal pain on the right side of the abdomen, just below the ribcage, with radiation of pain to the shoulder is classic.

Medicated aromatherapy bath – Bergamot, Chamomile and Geranium oil are all very good at easing the discomfort and for reducing the frequency of attacks. A warm medicated bath should be taken two or three times a week.

■ Abdominal colic, Diverticular Disease and Irritable Bowel Syndrome

Abdominal colic is the type of pain common in Diverticular disease of the colon (where there are small balloon-like swellings on the large bowel) and in Irritable Bowel Syndrome (where the bowel goes into variable spasm). All of these can be helped by various types of Sitz bath.

Hot Sitz bath – a short hot Sitz bath (see Chapter 3) is often very good at easing the acute pain of a severe attack of bowel spasm from either Diverticular Disease or Irritable Bowel Syndrome.

Medicated herbal Sitz bath – here an infusion of either Chamomile, Lavender or Peppermint is added to the main part of the warm bath. One soaks for twenty minutes or so.

Medicated aromatherapy Sitz bath – Bergamot, Black Pepper, Chamomile, Lavender, Marjoram or Peppermint oils can be added to the main part of the warm bath. Again, one soaks for twenty minutes or so.

■ Cystitis and urinary problems

Frequent passage of small quantities of urine together with a burning sensation as it is passed characterises Cystitis. It should be investigated by a health adviser swiftly, lest it develop into an ascending urinary infection to affect the kidneys. Antibiotics may be necessary, but as a first aid measure barley water can relieve the symptoms of burning.

A handful of pearl barley is scalded in a pint of boiling water and simmered for twenty minutes. It is then strained and flavoured with lemon juice. A tumblerful three times a day should bring symptomatic relief.

Contrast Sitz baths – if on a daily basis during the troubled time hot and cold Sitz baths are alternated, as described in Chapter 3, then the symptoms can be significantly eased.

Medicated herbal Sitz bath – Chamomile and Lavender infusions in a warm Sitz bath can prove very beneficial and soothing.

Medicated aromatherapy Sitz bath – Juniper, Sandalwood, or Tea-tree oil in a warm Sitz bath are all usually very soothing.

■ Bed-wetting

This condition always needs to be investigated to make sure that there is not a correctable cause. Once that has been excluded then the following may help.

Cold Sitz bath – this can help if one is taken on a daily basis. It should not be given to very young children, however. This is because it could be regarded as a punitive measure (which it isn't). The potential harm that this would sub-consciously do would make the whole thing counter-productive.

Medicated aromatherapy Sitz bath – Cypress oil seems to work very well with many children who have this problem. If they are unhappy about taking a Sitz bath, then an ordinary medicated bath will suffice.

■ Prostate problems

The prostate gland commonly enlarges about the age of sixty in men. When it does so it often produces a slowing down of the urinary stream, loss of power of the stream, a tendency to dribble after passing urine, and a tendency to have to get up in the night to pass urine.

These symptoms have to be investigated, since Cancer of the prostate can present in exactly the same way. It is treatable, provided that there is no delay in diagnosis.

Pumpkin seed and Sunflower seeds are worth eating as part of the regular diet, since both seem to have a beneficial effect upon the gland.

Retention enema – a slightly warm infusion of Chamomile is drawn up into the tube of a small bulb enema syringe (see Chapter 3) and gently squeezed into the rectum at night. This is then retained for as long as possible, if possible until the next bowel movement. Often this will directly ease the prostate bed.

Contrast Sitz baths – (see Chapter 3) If these are taken on a daily basis then there is a good chance that one might be able to alleviate the troublesome night-time problem.

Medicated herbal Sitz bath – Chamomile or Lemon balm infusions in the hot part of the medicated Sitz bath can help with prostatic symptoms.

Medicated aromatherapy Sitz bath – Jasmine and Juniper oils are the treatments of choice.

■ Male impotence

This can take several forms, including erectile impotence, ejaculatory failure or premature ejaculation. A medical opinion is always worth seeking.

Cold Sitz baths twice a week with a *Salt glow* twice a week (on different days from the Sitz baths) will often produce a good effect.

■ Constipation

A sudden change in bowel habit must always be investigated, so that serious conditions of the colon or rectum can be excluded.

Provided one has a good wholesome diet with plenty of dietary fibre then there should be little need for laxatives. In general, if someone is at the point of requiring suppositories or purgative enemas then they are at a point where they require a medical opinion.

Medicated herbal Sitz bath – Chamomile, Dandelion or Fennel in the warm part of a Sitz bath, three times a week should help many cases of constipation due to sluggish motility of the large bowel.

Medicated aromatherapy Sitz bath – Black Pepper, Chamomile, Fennel, Marjoram or Rose oil in a Sitz bath, three times a week.

■ Haemorrhoids

These are varicose veins of the rectum. They can itch, bleed or just be uncomfortable if they protrude from the rectum. A good wholesome diet with plenty of fibre is important to prevent straining when opening the bowels.

Medicated Sitz bath – this is helpful when there are prolapsed (protruding) acutely painful haemorrhoids. It is helpful to sit on a soft pad at the bottom of a bath which has Cypress, Geranium or Juniper oil added.

If there is very acute pain, then a Cold Sitz bath with one of these oils might help.

CHAPTER NINE

Women's Problems

The menstrual cycle and the menopause can both affect the well-being of females in various ways. Hydrotherapy and the use of different bath agents can help greatly with common problems experienced during both the reproductive and the post-reproductive parts of a woman's life.

As with most abdominal and pelvic problems the Sitz bath really comes into its own.

■ Painful periods

Dysmenorrhoea is the medical term for painful periods. It is something which most women will experience during some part of their reproductive life. If it persists over several periods then a medical opinion is indicated.

In young women under the age of 25 years the cause of the pain is often simply spasm. In older women it could be due to endometriosis, chronic pelvic inflammatory disease, ovarian cysts or the twisting of small fibroids.

Medicated herbal Sitz bath – Chamomile, Lavender or Rose infusions in a warm Sitz bath every other day from mid-cycle onwards can often ease the developing pelvic congestion as one approaches the period.

Medicated aromatherapy Sitz bath – Chamomile, Clary Sage, Cypress, Lavender, Marjoram or Rosemary oils in a warm Sitz bath taken every other day, as with the herbal bath can prevent painful periods.

Contrast Sitz bath – a warm-hot Sitz bath during the pain, deep enough to actually get the abdomen and pelvis submerged will often ease off the acute pain at the start of the period. This should be alternated with a lukewarm Sitz bath, as described in Chapter 3.

■ Heavy periods

This is often a subjective assessment on the part of the woman herself. A sudden change in the pattern of one's periods should always be treated seriously and a medical opinion be sought.

Medicated aromatherapy Sitz bath – Chamomile, Cypress, Geranium or Rose oils in a warm Sitz bath, every other day from mid-cycle onwards can often ease up the amount of the menstrual flow.

■ Pre-menstrual Syndrome (PMS)

This condition has three components – emotional, physical and behavioural. Usually the problem starts from the middle of the cycle and continues until the period has finished.

Most women experience some premenstrual symptoms at some stage. Some 30-40 per cent will have sufficient trouble to seek medical aid, while 5 per cent will find life so difficult that they will not be able to function for several days each month.

The commonest symptoms are:-

Emotional – depression, anxiety, irritability, hostility, jealousy, weepiness and indifference.

Physical – abdominal bloating, breast bloating, neck bloating, headache, fluid retention and acne.

Behavioural – aggression, avoidance of others, altered sex drive and pattern, depression.

Medicated herbal Sitz bath – Chamomile, Lavender or Rose infusions in a warm Sitz bath every other day from mid-cycle.

Medicated aromatherapy Sitz bath – Chamomile, Cypress, Geranium, Lavender, Marjoram or Rose oils in a warm Sitz bath every other day from mid-cycle.

■ Subfertility

Fertility has been one of the main concerns for people in every society. For some people the worry about not conceiving and producing a family can totally dominate their lives. If a couple have not conceived after about eight months of unprotected intercourse then they should seek medical advice.

Very often no reason for the failure to conceive can be found. It may be that for some reason there is just too much pelvic congestion. Or there may just be too much tension.

The couple should aim at making love at least twice, but no more often than three times a week. After every love-making the woman should rest in bed for about an hour, with the bottom end of the bed slightly raised (about 2 inches) on books.

1) Salt glow – a regular weekly Salt glow (as described in Chapter 3) should be taken by each of the partners. They should retire to a warm bed and make no attempt at love-making. A detoxification reaction is intended.

The above should be combined with:-

2) Medicated aromatherapy bath – A Sitz bath three times a week is recommended The first bath should be taken with Geranium, the second with Rose and the third one with Ylang Ylang.

3) A cup of Ginseng on three nights a week is advised.

■ Vaginal discharge

(see Chapter 10)

■ The Menopause

The menopause can be a traumatic problem for many women. It marks the cessation of the reproductive life, so it is a time of great change. There are alterations in hormonal levels as the ovaries stop producing eggs, there is a loss of bone substance (possibly actually resulting in osteoporosis) and there is a psychological adjustment to be made.

The main problem is the drop in the level of oestrogen. This directly causes flushing and vaginal dryness. This also contributes to the loss of calcium and to Osteoporosis. It is not known whether this directly causes some of the other symptoms, but it is likely that it is somehow involved.

Hormone Replacement treatment (HRT) has been a great boon to many women. Unfortunately, not everyone is able to tolerate it. Simple measures might help:-

1) Stop smoking
2) Take exercise which is reasonable for your age and degree of fitness.
3) Increase the calcium content of your diet. This means take plenty of dairy products, particularly yoghurt.
4) Take a phyto-oestrogen supplement. These are substances of plant origin which actually resemble oestrogen. Linseed oil (from Flax) is worth taking in capsule form (available from health shops) in a dose of two to five capsules a day. These will often significantly improve the vaginal dryness of the menopause.

Cold Sitz baths – these are taken regularly twice every week. They can help flushes. Avoid hot baths, since these will provoke the flushing.

Medicated herbal Sitz baths – these should be taken with lukewarm water, so as not to provoke the flushing. Chamomile, Lavender and Jasmine all seem to help.

Medicated aromatherapy Sitz baths – these also should be taken with lukewarm water. Chamomile, Cypress, Fennel, Geranium, Jasmine, Lavender and Rose oils are all of value in bringing relief.

PREGNANCY

Pregnancy is obviously not a problem in itself, yet there are many troublesome things that can ruin a woman's sense of well-being when she is pregnant.

Pregnancy is usually thought of as being composed of three Trimesters, each of about 13 weeks duration. The first Trimester is a vulnerable time which may be characterised by Nausea. The mid-Trimester is usually the time when a woman feels best, having gotten over the early Nausea. The features of the third Trimester include the continued increase in size of the womb, the softening of ligaments and the loss of mobility which results.

The less medication that one takes during pregnancy the better. A good wholesome, balanced diet, ensuring plenty of the essential vitamins and iron is more important. In addition, the bath can be a source of great benefit in those forty weeks.

■ Morning sickness

This can be extremely debilitating, at its worst turning into the condition of *hyperemesis gravidarum*, wherein the woman cannot even keep fluids down. Hospitalisation may be necessary on occasions.

71

Medicated aromatherapy bath – Ginger or Lavender oils are usually very helpful in a bath every other day.

■ Pregnancy tiredness

As the pregnancy advances most women feel tired. In part this can be due to a falling haemoglobin, but it is likely that part of the problem is the fluctuation in hormonal levels.

Medicated herbal bath – an infusion of Lavender is often refreshing.

Medicated aromatherapy bath – Grapefruit or Mandarin oils are refreshing.

POSTNATAL

■ Bruising

Medicated aromatherapy Sitz bath – after the birth of the baby the feeling of bruising in the perineum can be eased by taking Lavender in a lukewarm-warm medicated aromatherapy Sitz bath.

■ Breast feeding

Medicated aromatherapy bath – the flow of milk can be helped by Fennel or Geranium oils in a lukewarm-warm bath.

CHAPTER TEN

Troublesome Infections

So, naturalists observe, a flea
Hath smaller fleas that on him prey;
And these have smaller fleas to bite 'em,
And so proceed *ad infinitum.*
                    JOHNATHAN SWIFT 1667–1745

Many people go through life suffering from recurrent infections of the skin, urinary tract, bowel and genital tract. Trips to doctors and specialists do not seem to improve matters. Again, help may be found in the humble bath and appropriate types of douche, spray and bath additive.

■ The body's natural microbial partnership

It is a fact that the body is covered from the top of the head to the tip of the toe by a number of microbes. Back in 1674 Anton van Leeuwenhoek, a Dutch cloth merchant and dabbler in science, manufactured a microscope so powerful that he was the first man to see bacteria and microbes. After examining a specimen of scrapings from his own teeth he reported:

'I then saw, with great wonder. . many very little animalcules, very prettily a-moving.'

Over the years the science of microbiology grew up. It became clear that beyond the naked eye there is a veritable microbial jungle. Some of the microbes are beneficial to man and others are opportunistic invaders which can wreak great harm, cause countless infections and even bring about death.

Generally speaking, humans need their personal microbes. Some skin bacteria digest sebaceous fluid to produce useful protective germicidal chemicals. The female vagina is colonised by *Döderleins bacillus*, a specific lacto-bacillus. The large bowel has a large reservoir of commensal bacteria which helps the digestive tract to break down foods and waste products of digestion. All of these are beneficial to the body.

Sometimes, for one reason or another (such as the presence of a disease like Diabetes Mellitus, or an immune deficiency state) the commensal bacteria (natural microbes of the body) are displaced by a microbe which is completely parasitic. When this happens an infection may get a foothold. Sometimes that foothold is extremely hard to break.

When the body is subject to a persistent chronic infection then it may be that there is a hidden reservoir of the infecting organism somewhere on the body. The nose, for example, is one of the commonest sites for an individual to carry *Staphylococcus aureus*, a bacteria responsible for many chronic skin infections.

■ Skin infections

When there is a persistent skin infection then it is sensible to seek a medical opinion and medical treatment. The following measures can, however, prove helpful in the overall management.

Nasal douche – as mentioned above, nasal carriage of infecting bacteria is common in people prone to recurrent skin troubles, such as:- leg Ulcers, Impetigo, severe Acne, infected Eczema and other secondarily infected skin conditions.

A moderate infusion of Echinacea, or even weak cold tea can be effectively taken as a nasal douche every day for a week to eradicate such a source (see Chapter 3). A salt water douche, made by adding a teaspoon of salt to a pint of boiled, then cooled water, is also often effective.

Salt glow – this is an excellent way of provoking a detoxification and perspiration reaction. It should be taken as in Chapter 3, but it should not be used over areas of broken skin, or on weeping skin lesions.

Salt bath – a warm medicated salt bath is useful in dealing with many chronic skin infections. It should be taken twice a week.

Peat and peloid baths – a full peat bath is difficult to use in the home, but a modified one with liquid peat extract (see Chapter 3) can be extremely good at dealing with troublesome skin infections. It should be taken twice a week until improvement begins.

Mud packs – mud from Neydharting is obtainable from many health shops. It contains natural antibiotic agents and can, therefore, be used beneficially as a local body pack over a specific area of infected Eczema (see Chapter 3).

Medicated herbal bath – Echinacea, or tea and salt combined in a warm bath are often highly effective at improving infective skin conditions.

Medicated aromatherapy bath – Lavender, Patchouli, Tea-tree and Thyme oils are all very good for dealing with troublesome bacterial skin infections.

Cold showers – with most skin infections the application of heat tends to stimulate the infection. Conversely, the application of cold water under pressure tends to inhibit microbial activity. Therefore, when treating any skin infection it is a good idea to use a hand spray or hand shower after the treatment.

■ Ringworm, Athlete's Foot and other fungal infections

Athlete's foot, ringworm and most of the common skin fungal infections are caused by tineal fungi which are capable of digesting keratin. Keratin is the horny layer of the skin and the substance of hair and nails.

Impetigo is an infection caused by a yeast-like fungus, *Candida albicans*, which is common in the groins, in skinfolds and under the breasts in women.

Salt foot or partial body baths (if possible) — salt foot baths three times a week are good for easing Athlete's foot and other localised fungal infections.

Peat and peloid partial body baths — see above. These foot baths using liquid peat extract can be extremely good at dealing with difficult fungal infections. They should be taken twice or three times a week until improvement begins.

Medicated aromatherapy baths — Lavender, Myrrh, Patchouli or Tea-tree oils are very helpful in dealing with many fungal infections.

■ Vaginal infections

Irritation of the vulva and vagina, with or without a vaginal discharge is extremely common.

As mentioned above *Döderleins bacillus* is the normal bacteria that inhabits the female front passage. Antibiotics taken for an infection somewhere else in the body frequently cause a reduction in the number of *Döderleins bacilli* and effectively open the door for an opportunistic infection by an organism such as *Candida albicans* — commonly called *thrush*.

Many couples find that one or both of them tends to keep getting infected. Usually, it is the woman who ends up with a white, irritant vaginal discharge.

One of the problems, and one of the misleading factors, is the observation that men tend not to have many symptoms. Indeed, they may never seem to have the problem. The reality, however, is that they are usually the ones to harbour the infection.

Candida albicans exists in both a spore phase and a vegetative phase. When it is actively thriving in the vegetative phase, it exists in a form which results in obvious lesions. The infected membranes appear red and angry and white flecks are visible. In a woman there is usually a discharge. The spore phase is a dormant and protected phase. It is in this form that men often harbour the organism, either under their foreskin or deep inside their bodies, in the seminal vesicles.

Unprotected intercourse produces the correct conditions of moisture, heat and friction for the transfer of the spores and their subsequent reactivation and growth. The subsequent development of symptoms can happen with great rapidity.

The spores are the problem. They are capable of withstanding extreme conditions. They survive in flannels, sponges and loofahs for days, weeks and possibly months. Similarly, they can dry up and survive in underclothes.

One can see how this can be a problem. Most people use bath flannels, sponges, etc. Unfortunately they can literally act as a breeding ground to a number of organisms. In my opinion they should be used relatively rarely in the bathroom or shower, and they should never be used to wash and cleanse the nether regions!

Boiling of clothes, flannels etc is the best way of getting rid of candida spores, if one cannot afford to jettison them! And after they have been boiled for a long time, they should be hung up to dry in the sun. The ultra-violet rays of the sun are also deleterious to the candida spores.

Although I have been talking about Candida albicans above, the following remedies should help most vaginal infections.

Salt baths – these are often very effective in easing the intense itch of thrush, since they produce an environment hostile to the organism. They should not be taken hot, but should be lukewarm.

Medicated herbal bath – Chamomile, Echinacea and tea infusions in a lukewarm bath, twice a day for several days may ease a current infection. They can help prevent recurrence if taken once or twice a week.

Medicated aromatherapy bath – Bergamot, Lavender, Lemon and Tea-tree oils are all helpful in dealing with acute infections and recurrences of thrush.

Vaginal douches – an infusion of Chamomile, tea or Lavender used in a scrupulously clean vaginal douche (see Chapter 3) twice a day will usually give symptomatic improvement and start to get rid of a thrush or other vaginal infection.

■ Recurrent urinary infections

Troublesome urinary infections plague some people's lives. While one cannot directly reach the urinary tract one can help recurrent infections by external hydrotherapeutic techniques.

The presence of a kidney or bladder stone or lesion might act as a focus of infection, thereby leading to recurrent problems. By stimulating the skin's excretory role, through a perspiration and detoxification reaction one can aid the kidney by removing some of the strain upon it.

Epsom Salt bath – taking such a bath once a fortnight can often help reduce the frequency of attacks of urinary infections. One should only contemplate this if one is fairly fit and does not suffer from a heart problem, kidney failure or disease, or hypertension.

Hot plain bath – a weekly bath at 100°–107°F (38°–41°C) for ten minutes, followed by a swift cold hand-showering.

Partial body wraps – these are mini-versions of the whole body wrap. If one is used around the trunk then a reasonable perspiration reaction can be induced. Again, this is worth doing every fortnight (see Chapter 3).

Medicated aromatherapy Sitz bath – Lavender, Juniper, Sandalwood and Tea-tree oils are useful in helping prevent recurrent urinary infections.

■ Bowel infections

Diarrhoea is one of the main symptoms of bowel infection. It is absolutely imperative, however, that one should seek medical advice if there is an alteration of one's bowel habit which does not settle within days. Cancer of the bowel is too important a condition to delay diagnosis.

Medicated aromatherapy Sitz bath – Bergamot, Black pepper, Chamomile, Geranium, Lavender, Rosemary and Sandalwood oils are all potentially very good for helping to settle diarrhoeal illnesses down.

■ Anal fissures and pilonidal sinuses

These are tears around the back passage, or around hair follicles near to the anus. They can be excruciatingly painful.

Salt baths – these will sting, but they do tend to resolve the inflammation associated with these problems.

Medicated aromatherapy bath – Lavender or Tea-tree oils are both very helpful in soothing these problems.

CHAPTER ELEVEN

Troubled Emotions

Most people are aware of the relaxing effect of a good warm bath and of the stimulating effect of a cold shower. These are simple examples of the way in which water can affect the way we feel. Yet there is much greater scope than this. The appropriate type of bath, technique and bath additive can help ease insomnia, anxiety and lowered spirits.

■ Anxiety

At some stage or another everyone will feel anxious. It is part of life. When faced with a situation which you find threatening, be that physically or psychologically, then the body responds by creating the experience of anxiety.

All emotions are hard to define, but you can come close when you look at them in terms of three components – physical, psychological and behavioural.

Taking anxiety as an example, the adrenal gland pumps out adrenaline which causes the sympathetic nervous system to speed up the heart, quicken the breathing and dilate the pupils. This is the physical part.

The psychological part comes when the mind conceptualises the experience of this physical sensation in the face of the stimulus. If it is perceived as being unpleasant then the sensation of anxiety deepens.

Finally, the behavioural response is governed by whether the mind allows the individual to face up to the situation or choose to 'run for it.'

This is a very simplistic analysis of anxiety and fear. The fact is that fear and anxiety can be helped by doing things which help to lower the threshold of adrenaline release and which induce a relaxation response. Various types of bath can do this.

Hot bath – a hot bath last thing at night induces, as you know, a relaxation response. It also may tend to set off a perspiration reaction, so one should generally not go out after having one.

Medicated herbal bath – an infusion of Chamomile, Lavender or Gentian are all very useful in inducing a relaxation feeling.

Medicated aromatherapy bath – Chamomile, Jasmine, Sandalwood and Ylang Ylang are all extremely helpful for conditions of anxiety.

■ Depression

Most people feel sad at times in their lives. Sometimes there seems to be an obvious trigger or series of provoking factors. And sometimes it just seems that a black dog has jumped on your back.

The features of being significantly depressed include:-

- lowness of spirits
- loss of vitality
- feelings of guilt
- self depreciation
- hopelessness and despair
- sleep disturbance
- variation in mood throughout the day
- thoughts of self harm

The more of these factors that one feels the greater is the need to seek help. There is no need to feel embarrassed about this, since feelings are part of being human. Although you may usually be able to pull yourself out of the blues, sometimes you may need help.

Medicated herbal bath – Chamomile, Gentian and Valerian are all worth considering putting in the bath when there is mild depression.

Medicated aromatherapy bath – Basil, Bergamot, Chamomile, Jasmine, Lavender, Rose, Sandalwood, Thyme and Ylang Ylang are all of value in mild depression.

■ Insomnia

Insomnia is a blanket description for all sorts of sleep disturbance. It is actually common at all ages. Some people equate it with lack of sleep time, others with difficulty getting off to sleep, and still others with a tendency to wake repeatedly.

The best working definition I know of is that insomnia is a difficulty in initiating and/or maintaining sleep which is satisfying.

Hot bath – as mentioned above, a hot bath at night is often enough to help someone get off to sleep by its tendency to induce a relaxation response.

Medicated herbal bath – Chamomile, Lavender, and Rose infusions in a bath every other night may well help with insomnia.

Medicated aromatherapy bath – Chamomile, Lavender, Rose, Sandalwood and Ylang Ylang are all effective for easing insomnia.

■ Chronic Fatigue Syndrome

This condition or symptom cluster has come to prominence over the last few years. It is another blanket description for a whole range of conditions, all of which have chronic exhaustion as one of their main symptoms and features.

Myalgic Encephalomyelitis (ME), 'Yuppie Flu', Post Viral Syndrome are three examples of the labels that have been used to describe the problem. They all have different implications. ME implies that it is a condition with a real physical and neurological basis. Yuppie Flu is a disparaging, non-believing and cruel description. Finally, Post Viral Syndrome is a grudging acceptance of a state of exhaustion following a viral infection of some sort.

The fact is that the Chronic Fatigue Syndrome is very real. It causes a lot of problems for people because they just cannot summon enough energy to cope with their normal daily activities. It imposes a lot of pressure upon the individual and upon the individual's family.

While hydrotherapy cannot produce any sort of a cure for this problem it can help. It is important, however to ensure that the type of baths and showers are stimulating and not sedative. Indeed, too many hot baths and showers will do nothing but help to deplete the individual's vitality.

Medicated herbal Sitz bath – Lavender in the warm part of the Sitz bath seems to be quite helpful when there is low vitality.

Medicated aromatherapy bath – Clary Sage, Eucalyptus, Juniper and Thyme are all stimulating.

Mustard foot bath – taking a mustard foot bath twice a week is beneficial for the aching legs which are commonly complained of in this syndrome.

■ **Anger**

People feel angry at various times in their lives. It is an emotion which can be very destructive to the individual if it is permitted to continue without being calmed. Just think of the expressions associated with it – 'red with anger', 'white with rage', 'blood boiling,' plus many others. The significance of these is that this emotion does affect one's circulation. If allowed to persist it can have dire consequences.

Medicated herbal bath – Chamomile, Lavender or Gentian are all very useful in helping to reduce one's anger. The temperature of the bath should only be tepid.

Medicated aromatherapy bath – Chamomile and Ylang Ylang are good for soothing anger.

■ Grief

Hardly anyone goes through life without experiencing the pangs of grief. It is part of being human.

Three stages of grief are well recognised:-

1) Shock – this lasts for a week or two. It is the mind's way of lessening the pain.
2) Intense grief and distress – this lasts up to three months. During this time it is common to experience anger, guilt, depression and anxiety.
3) Continued depression – this can last for another three months.

These stages represent 'normal grief.' Some people may suffer intensely for considerably longer, but as a rule of thumb most people should be experiencing some softening of the emotional pain by six months. If there is no improvement then a medical opinion is indicated.

Medicated aromatherapy baths – I find that these often help considerably. In particular, Frankincense, Marjoram, Neroli and Rose work well.

■ Jealousy

This emotion is hardly ever considered seriously by the medical profession, yet it is another fearfully destructive emotion. The green-eyed monster of jealousy can destroy lives.

Medicated aromatherapy bath – soaking in a Rose essential oil bath twice or three times a week can work wonders on this emotion.

■ Anorexia nervosa

Body image and eating disorders are conditions which must have an early medical opinion.

Medicated aromatherapy baths – Basil, Benzoin, Jasmine, Lavender, Sandalwood, Thyme and Ylang Ylang may all individually help if taken in a bath twice a week.